HEART HEALTHY FOODS CHART

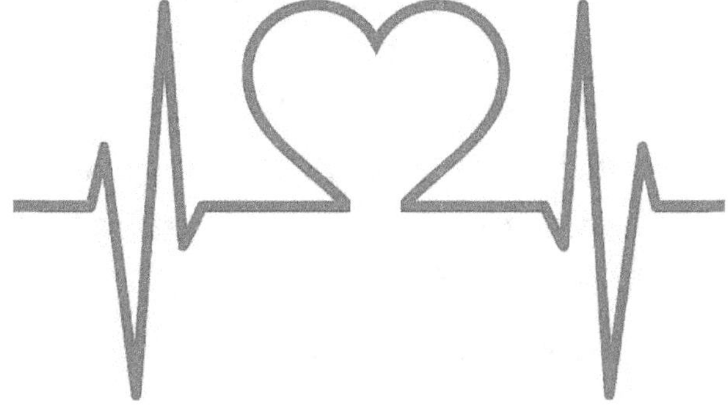

Unlock the secrets to optimal cardiovascular health with a visually engaging chart showcasing nutrient-rich foods and empowering you to make heart-conscious dietary decisions

Felicia O. Pace

TABLE OF CONTENTS

INTRODUCTION

Ensuring a heart-healthy lifestyle is paramount for overall well-being, and one of the foundational pillars of cardiovascular health is a nutritious diet. The Heart Healthy Foods Chart serves as a valuable tool to guide individuals towards making informed and health-conscious choices in their dietary habits. This chart is designed to highlight foods that are not only delicious but also promote heart health by incorporating essential nutrients, antioxidants, and fiber while minimizing harmful elements such as saturated fats, sodium, and added sugars.

In the journey towards cardiovascular wellness, the Heart Healthy Foods Chart serves as a visual roadmap, offering a comprehensive overview of foods that can contribute to a heart-healthy diet. It emphasizes the significance of balance, diversity, and portion control, showcasing a variety of nutrient-rich options across different food groups. Whether you are aiming to prevent heart disease, manage existing conditions, or simply adopt a healthier lifestyle, this chart provides a user-friendly reference to support your dietary choices.

The Heart Healthy Foods Chart is a dynamic resource that can be tailored to individual preferences, cultural considerations, and dietary needs. It not only encourages the consumption of heart-protective foods but also raises awareness about those that should be limited or avoided to maintain optimal cardiovascular health. As we embark on this journey towards heart wellness, let the Heart Healthy Foods Chart be your companion, offering insights, inspiration, and practical guidance to foster a lifetime of heart-healthy eating habits.

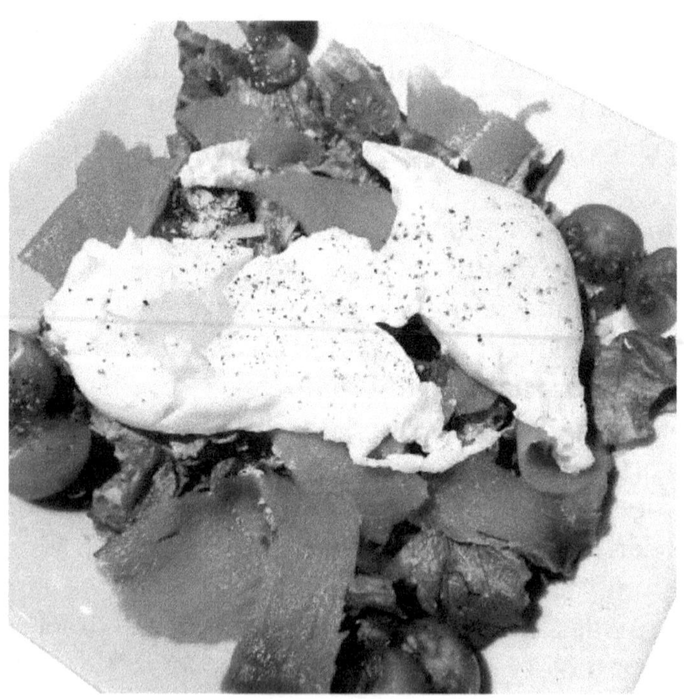

Heart Healthy meal planning Tips

Heart-healthy meal planning is an essential component of managing heart health and reducing the risk of cardiovascular diseases. Here are extensive tips to help you plan and enjoy heart-healthy meals:

1. Focus on Whole Foods:
   - Prioritize whole, unprocessed foods like fruits, vegetables, whole grains, lean proteins, and healthy fats.
   - Choose colorful fruits and vegetables, as they are rich in antioxidants and essential nutrients.

2. Choose Heart-Healthy Fats:
   - Opt for sources of unsaturated fats such as olive oil, avocados, nuts, and seeds.
   - Limit saturated and trans fats found in processed foods, fried foods, and certain animal products.

3. Include Omega-3 Fatty Acids:
   - Incorporate fatty fish (salmon, mackerel, sardines) at least twice a week.
   - Include flaxseeds, chia seeds, and walnuts, which are plant-based sources of omega-3s.

4. Limit Sodium Intake:
- Reduce the use of table salt and choose herbs, spices, and other seasonings to flavor dishes.
- Be mindful of processed foods, as they often contain high levels of hidden sodium.

5. Choose Lean Proteins:
- Opt for lean protein sources like skinless poultry, lean cuts of meat, fish, tofu, legumes, and low-fat dairy.
- Limit red meat and processed meats, as they may contribute to heart disease.

6. Incorporate Fiber-Rich Foods:
- Include whole grains, legumes, fruits, and vegetables to boost fiber intake.
- Fiber helps lower cholesterol levels and promotes a healthy digestive system.

7. Portion Control:
- Pay attention to portion sizes to avoid overeating, which can contribute to weight gain and heart issues.
- Use smaller plates and bowls to help control portion sizes.

8. Plan Balanced Meals:
- Create balanced meals that include a variety of food groups – vegetables, fruits, whole grains, proteins, and healthy fats.
- Aim for a diverse range of colors on your plate to ensure a mix of nutrients.

9. Cook at Home:
- Prepare meals at home to have better control over ingredients and cooking methods.
- Experiment with heart-healthy recipes to make cooking enjoyable.

10. Mindful Eating:
- Practice mindful eating by savoring each bite and paying attention to hunger and fullness cues.
- Avoid distractions like TV or electronic devices during meals.

11. Stay Hydrated:
- Drink plenty of water throughout the day to stay hydrated.
- Limit sugary drinks and excessive caffeine intake.

12. Limit Added Sugars:
   - Reduce consumption of sugary snacks, desserts, and sweetened beverages.
   - Opt for natural sweeteners like honey or maple syrup in moderation.

13. Meal Prep and Planning:
   - Plan your meals and snacks in advance to ensure a well-balanced diet.
   - Prepare and portion meals ahead of time to make healthy choices more convenient.

14. Read Food Labels:
   - Check nutrition labels for sodium, saturated fats, and added sugars.
   - Choose products with minimal processing and additives.

15. Regular Physical Activity:
   - Combine heart-healthy eating with regular physical activity for overall cardiovascular health.
   - Aim for at least 150 minutes of moderate-intensity exercise per week.

16. Consult a Registered Dietitian:
- Seek advice from a registered dietitian or healthcare professional for personalized guidance based on your health needs and goals.

Food to limit or avoid

Maintaining a heart-healthy diet involves not only incorporating nutrient-rich foods but also being mindful of those that can contribute to heart disease. Here's an extensive overview of foods to limit or avoid for heart health:

1. Saturated and Trans Fats:
- Limit: Red meat, full-fat dairy products, processed meats (sausages, bacon), fried foods, and commercially baked goods.
- Why: High consumption of saturated and trans fats can raise LDL (bad) cholesterol levels, contributing to heart disease.

2. Excessive Sodium:
- Limit: Processed foods, canned soups, salty snacks, and high-sodium condiments.
- Why: Excess sodium can lead to high blood pressure, increasing the risk of heart disease and stroke.

3. Added Sugars:
   - Limit: Sugary beverages, candies, pastries, and processed foods with added sugars.
   - Why: Diets high in added sugars can contribute to obesity, diabetes, and heart disease.

4. Processed and Packaged Foods:
   - Avoid: Foods with high levels of additives, preservatives, and artificial ingredients.
   - Why: Processed foods often contain unhealthy fats, excess sodium, and added sugars, impacting heart health.

5. Highly Processed Carbohydrates:
   - Limit: White bread, white rice, and sugary cereals.
   - Why: Refined carbohydrates can contribute to weight gain and increase the risk of heart disease.

6. Limit Alcohol Consumption:
   - Moderation: While moderate alcohol consumption may have heart benefits, excessive drinking can lead to high blood pressure and heart failure.
   - Why: Heavy alcohol consumption is associated with cardiovascular problems.

7. High-Caffeine and Energy Drinks:
   - Limit: Beverages with excessive caffeine content.
   - Why: High caffeine intake may lead to irregular heartbeats and increased blood pressure in some individuals.

8. Avoid Trans Fats:
   - Avoid: Foods containing partially hydrogenated oils.
   - Why: Trans fats raise LDL cholesterol levels and lower HDL (good) cholesterol, contributing to heart disease.

9. Limit Red Meat and Processed Meats:
   - Limit: Beef, pork, and processed meats like hot dogs and sausages.
   - Why: High consumption of red and processed meats is linked to heart disease.

10. Fried Foods:
   - Limit: Fried foods like French fries, fried chicken, and doughnuts.
   - Why: Fried foods can be high in unhealthy fats, contributing to high cholesterol and heart disease.

11. Limit Full-Fat Dairy:
   - Limit: Whole milk, full-fat cheese, and butter.
   - Why: High saturated fat content in full-fat dairy products can raise cholesterol levels.

12. Highly Processed Cooking Oils:
   - Limit: Cooking oils high in trans fats or saturated fats, like palm oil.
   - Why:Opt for heart-healthy oils such as olive oil or canola oil.

13. Limit Fast Food:
   - Limit: Fast food items that are often high in unhealthy fats, sodium, and calories.
   - Why: Regular consumption of fast food is associated with an increased risk of heart disease.

14. Avoid Excessive Caloric Intake:
   - Moderation: Be mindful of portion sizes to avoid excessive caloric intake.
   - Why: Obesity is a major risk factor for heart disease.

15. High-Cholesterol Foods:
   - Limit: Shellfish, organ meats, and high-cholesterol animal products.
   - Why: High-cholesterol foods can contribute to elevated blood cholesterol levels.

Fruits

Berry Smoothie Bowl:
Ingredients: Mixed berries (strawberries, blueberries, raspberries), low-fat yogurt, banana, chia seeds.
Nutritional Intake (per serving): Calories: 250, Fiber: 8g, Protein: 10g, Vitamin C: 80mg.

Citrus Salad with Mint:
Ingredients: Oranges, grapefruits, mint leaves.
Nutritional Intake (per serving): Calories: 120, Fiber: 5g, Vitamin C: 70mg.

Kiwi and Spinach Salad:
Ingredients: Kiwi, spinach, almonds, feta cheese.
Nutritional Intake (per serving): Calories: 180, Fiber: 6g, Vitamin K: 150mcg.

Mango Salsa:
Ingredients: Mango, red onion, cilantro, lime juice.
Nutritional Intake (per serving): Calories: 80, Vitamin A: 1000IU, Vitamin C: 45mg.

Baked Apples with Cinnamon:
Ingredients: Apples, cinnamon, a touch of honey.
Nutritional Intake (per serving): Calories: 100, Fiber: 4g, Vitamin C: 10mg.

Pineapple and Avocado Salad:
Ingredients: Pineapple, avocado, cherry tomatoes, lime juice.
Nutritional Intake (per serving): Calories: 160, Fiber: 7g, Vitamin C: 40mg.

Blueberry Oat Muffins:
Ingredients: Blueberries, oats, whole wheat flour, Greek yogurt.
Nutritional Intake (per serving): Calories: 150, Fiber: 5g, Protein: 8g.

Papaya and Lime Sorbet:
Ingredients: Papaya, lime juice, a touch of agave syrup.
Nutritional Intake (per serving): Calories: 120, Vitamin A: 1500IU, Vitamin C: 30mg.

Watermelon and Feta Salad:
Ingredients: Watermelon, feta cheese, mint leaves.
Nutritional Intake (per serving): Calories: 100, Vitamin A: 1000IU, Vitamin C: 20mg.

Chia Seed Pudding with Berries:
Ingredients: Chia seeds, almond milk, mixed berries.
Nutritional Intake (per serving): Calories: 180, Fiber: 10g, Protein: 5g.

Vegetables

Grilled Vegetable Skewers:
Ingredients: Bell peppers, cherry tomatoes, zucchini, red onion, olive oil.
Nutritional Intake (per serving): Calories: 120, Fiber: 6g, Vitamin C: 60mg.

Spinach and Mushroom Quinoa Bowl:
Ingredients: Spinach, mushrooms, quinoa, garlic, olive oil.
Nutritional Intake (per serving): Calories: 200, Fiber: 8g, Protein: 10g.

Roasted Brussels Sprouts with Balsamic Glaze:
Ingredients: Brussels sprouts, balsamic vinegar, olive oil.
Nutritional Intake (per serving): Calories: 100, Fiber: 6g, Vitamin C: 48mg.

Stir-Fried Broccoli and Tofu:
Ingredients: Broccoli, tofu, ginger, soy sauce.
Nutritional Intake (per serving): Calories: 150, Fiber: 7g, Protein: 12g.

Sweet Potato and Kale Hash:
Ingredients: Sweet potatoes, kale, onions, olive oil.
Nutritional Intake (per serving): Calories: 180, Fiber: 8g, Vitamin A: 20000IU.

Cucumber and Tomato Salad:
Ingredients: Cucumbers, tomatoes, red onion, feta cheese, olive oil.
Nutritional Intake (per serving): Calories: 90, Vitamin C: 15mg.

Zucchini Noodles with Pesto:
Ingredients: Zucchini noodles, cherry tomatoes, basil pesto.
Nutritional Intake (per serving): Calories: 130, Fiber: 5g, Vitamin C: 25mg.

Eggplant and Chickpea Stew:
Ingredients: Eggplant, chickpeas, tomatoes, garlic, olive oil.
Nutritional Intake (per serving): Calories: 160, Fiber: 9g, Protein: 8g.

Asparagus and Lemon Roast:
Ingredients: Asparagus, lemon, garlic, olive oil.
Nutritional Intake (per serving): Calories: 70, Fiber: 5g, Vitamin C: 20mg.

Carrot and Ginger Soup:
Ingredients: Carrots, ginger, onion, vegetable broth.
Nutritional Intake (per serving): Calories: 120, Fiber: 5g, Vitamin A: 15000IU.

Legumes

Chickpea Salad:
Ingredients: Chickpeas, cherry tomatoes, cucumber, red onion, olive oil.
Nutritional Intake (per serving): Calories: 180, Fiber: 8g, Protein: 7g.

Lentil and Vegetable Curry:
Ingredients: Lentils, mixed vegetables, tomatoes, curry spices.
Nutritional Intake (per serving): Calories: 220, Fiber: 12g, Protein: 15g.

Black Bean and Corn Salsa:
Ingredients: Black beans, corn, bell peppers, cilantro, lime juice.
Nutritional Intake (per serving): Calories: 150, Fiber: 9g, Protein: 7g.

Split Pea Soup:
Ingredients: Split peas, carrots, celery, onion, vegetable broth.
Nutritional Intake (per serving): Calories: 180, Fiber: 10g, Protein: 12g.

Hummus with Veggies:
Ingredients: Chickpeas, tahini, garlic, lemon juice, assorted vegetables for dipping.
Nutritional Intake (per serving): Calories: 120, Fiber: 5g, Protein: 4g.

Quinoa and Black Bean Stuffed Peppers:
Ingredients: Black beans, quinoa, bell peppers, tomatoes, spices.
Nutritional Intake (per serving): Calories: 200, Fiber: 8g, Protein: 10g.

Red Lentil and Spinach Dal:
Ingredients: Red lentils, spinach, tomatoes, curry spices.
Nutritional Intake (per serving): Calories: 220, Fiber: 14g, Protein: 12g.

Edamame and Brown Rice Bowl:
Ingredients: Edamame, brown rice, carrots, broccoli, soy sauce.
Nutritional Intake (per serving): Calories: 250, Fiber: 10g, Protein: 15g.

White Bean and Kale Soup:
Ingredients: Cannellini beans, kale, tomatoes, garlic, vegetable broth.
Nutritional Intake (per serving): Calories: 160, Fiber: 8g, Protein: 10g.

Chana Masala:
Ingredients: Garbanzo beans (chickpeas), tomatoes, onions, spices.
Nutritional Intake (per serving): Calories: 180, Fiber: 10g, Protein: 8g.

Lean protein

Grilled Chicken Breast with Lemon and Herbs:
Ingredients: Chicken breast, lemon, garlic, rosemary, olive oil.
Nutritional Intake (per serving): Calories: 200, Protein: 25g.

Baked Salmon with Dill and Lemon:
Ingredients: Salmon fillet, dill, lemon, olive oil.
Nutritional Intake (per serving): Calories: 250, Protein: 20g, Omega-3 fatty acids.

Turkey and Vegetable Stir-Fry:
Ingredients: Lean ground turkey, mixed vegetables, soy sauce, ginger.
Nutritional Intake (per serving): Calories: 220, Protein: 18g.

Quinoa and Blackened Shrimp Bowl:
Ingredients: Shrimp, quinoa, blackening seasoning, bell peppers.
Nutritional Intake (per serving): Calories: 230, Protein: 20g.

Grilled Tofu and Vegetable Skewers:
Ingredients: Extra-firm tofu, bell peppers, cherry tomatoes, balsamic glaze.
Nutritional Intake (per serving): Calories: 180, Protein: 15g.

Lemon Garlic Herb Baked Cod:
Ingredients: Cod fillet, lemon, garlic, herbs, olive oil.
Nutritional Intake (per serving): Calories: 180, Protein: 22g.

Lean Beef and Vegetable Stir-Fry:
Ingredients: Lean beef strips, broccoli, carrots, soy sauce.
Nutritional Intake (per serving): Calories: 250, Protein: 25g.

Mushroom and Spinach Egg White Omelette:
Ingredients: Egg whites, mushrooms, spinach, feta cheese.
Nutritional Intake (per serving): Calories: 150, Protein: 20g.

Grilled Turkey Burgers with Avocado:
Ingredients: Lean ground turkey, whole grain buns, avocado, lettuce.
Nutritional Intake (per serving): Calories: 220, Protein: 18g.

Baked Halibut with Tomato and Olive Salsa:
Ingredients: Halibut fillet, tomatoes, olives, basil, olive oil.
Nutritional Intake (per serving): Calories: 200, Protein: 24g.

Free fats or low dairy fat

Avocado and Tomato Salad:
Ingredients: Avocado, cherry tomatoes, red onion, cilantro, lime juice.
Nutritional Intake (per serving): Calories: 150, Healthy Fats: 10g, Fiber: 6g.

Olive Oil and Herb Roasted Vegetables:
Ingredients: Mixed vegetables (zucchini, bell peppers, cherry tomatoes), olive oil, herbs.
Nutritional Intake (per serving): Calories: 120, Healthy Fats: 8g, Fiber: 5g.

Salmon and Quinoa Bowl with Lemon-Dill Dressing:
Ingredients: Grilled salmon, quinoa, cucumber, lemon-dill dressing.
Nutritional Intake (per serving): Calories: 250, Healthy Fats: 12g, Protein: 20g.

Greek Yogurt Parfait with Nuts and Berries:
Ingredients: Greek yogurt, mixed berries, almonds, honey.
Nutritional Intake (per serving): Calories: 180, Healthy Fats: 8g, Protein: 15g.

Walnut and Spinach Pesto Pasta:
Ingredients: Whole wheat pasta, spinach, garlic, walnuts, olive oil.
Nutritional Intake (per serving): Calories: 220, Healthy Fats: 10g, Fiber: 8g.

Mashed Sweet Potatoes with Coconut Milk:
Ingredients: Sweet potatoes, coconut milk, cinnamon.
Nutritional Intake (per serving): Calories: 180, Healthy Fats: 6g, Fiber: 5g.

Quinoa Salad with Chickpeas and Tahini Dressing:
Ingredients: Quinoa, chickpeas, cherry tomatoes, cucumber, tahini.
Nutritional Intake (per serving): Calories: 230, Healthy Fats: 10g, Protein: 8g.

Lemon Herb Baked Chicken Breast:
Ingredients: Chicken breast, lemon, garlic, herbs, olive oil.
Nutritional Intake (per serving): Calories: 200, Healthy Fats: 8g, Protein: 25g.

Cauliflower Rice Stir-Fry with Tofu:
Ingredients: Cauliflower rice, tofu, mixed vegetables, sesame oil.
Nutritional Intake (per serving): Calories: 180, Healthy Fats: 9g, Protein: 15g.

Almond-Crusted Baked Cod:
Ingredients: Cod fillet, almonds, lemon zest, olive oil.
Nutritional Intake (per serving): Calories: 210, Healthy Fats: 12g, Protein: 20g.

Whole grains

Quinoa Salad with Vegetables:
Ingredients: Quinoa, cherry tomatoes, cucumber, red onion, feta cheese, olive oil.
Nutritional Intake (per serving): Calories: 220, Whole Grains: 40g, Fiber: 8g.

Brown Rice and Black Bean Bowl:
Ingredients: Brown rice, black beans, corn, avocado, salsa.
Nutritional Intake (per serving): Calories: 250, Whole Grains: 45g, Fiber: 10g, Protein: 8g.

Oatmeal with Mixed Berries:
Ingredients: Rolled oats, mixed berries, almond milk, chia seeds.
Nutritional Intake (per serving): Calories: 180, Whole Grains: 30g, Fiber: 6g.

Whole Wheat Pasta Primavera:
Ingredients: Whole wheat pasta, mixed vegetables, tomato sauce, olive oil.
Nutritional Intake (per serving): Calories: 240, Whole Grains: 40g, Fiber: 7g.

Barley and Vegetable Soup:
Ingredients: Barley, carrots, celery, onions, vegetable broth.
Nutritional Intake (per serving): Calories: 200, Whole Grains: 35g, Fiber: 8g.

Farro and Roasted Vegetable Salad:
Ingredients: Farro, roasted vegetables (bell peppers, zucchini, cherry tomatoes), balsamic vinaigrette.
Nutritional Intake (per serving): Calories: 220, Whole Grains: 40g, Fiber: 6g.

Buckwheat Pancakes with Blueberries:
Ingredients: Buckwheat flour, almond milk, blueberries, maple syrup.
Nutritional Intake (per serving): Calories: 180, Whole Grains: 25g, Fiber: 5g.

Millet-Stuffed Bell Peppers:
Ingredients: Millet, bell peppers, black beans, corn, salsa.
Nutritional Intake (per serving): Calories: 230, Whole Grains: 35g, Fiber: 9g, Protein: 7g.

Wild Rice and Mushroom Pilaf:
Ingredients: Wild rice, mushrooms, garlic, vegetable broth.
Nutritional Intake (per serving): Calories: 210, Whole Grains: 35g, Fiber: 7g.

Spelt Flour Banana Bread:
Ingredients: Spelt flour, ripe bananas, walnuts, cinnamon.
Nutritional Intake (per serving): Calories: 150, Whole Grains: 20g, Fiber: 4g.

Nuts and Seeds

Chia Seed Pudding:
Ingredients: Chia seeds, almond milk, berries, honey.
Nutritional Intake (per serving): Calories: 180, Omega-3 Fatty Acids, Fiber: 10g.

Mixed Nut Trail Mix:
Ingredients: Almonds, walnuts, pistachios, dark chocolate chips, dried cranberries.
Nutritional Intake (per serving): Calories: 200, Healthy Fats, Protein: 8g.

Greek Yogurt Parfait with Nuts and Berries:
Ingredients: Greek yogurt, mixed berries, almonds, chia seeds.
Nutritional Intake (per serving): Calories: 220, Protein: 15g, Healthy Fats.

Pumpkin Seed and Spinach Salad:
Ingredients: Pumpkin seeds, spinach, cherry tomatoes, feta cheese, balsamic vinaigrette.
Nutritional Intake (per serving): Calories: 180, Protein: 10g, Omega-3 Fatty Acids.

Almond-Crusted Baked Chicken:
Ingredients: Almond meal, chicken breast, herbs, olive oil.
Nutritional Intake (per serving): Calories: 250, Protein: 30g, Healthy Fats.

Flaxseed and Banana Smoothie:
Ingredients: Flaxseeds, banana, yogurt, almond milk.
Nutritional Intake (per serving): Calories: 200, Omega-3 Fatty Acids, Protein: 8g.

Cashew and Date Energy Bites:
Ingredients: Cashews, dates, coconut, vanilla extract.
Nutritional Intake (per serving): Calories: 150, Protein: 5g, Healthy Fats.

Sunflower Seed and Avocado Toast:
Ingredients: Whole grain bread, avocado, sunflower seeds, cherry tomatoes.
Nutritional Intake (per serving): Calories: 220, Healthy Fats, Fiber: 8g.

Walnut and Kale Pesto Pasta:
Ingredients: Walnuts, kale, garlic, whole wheat pasta, olive oil.
Nutritional Intake (per serving): Calories: 240, Omega-3 Fatty Acids, Fiber: 6g.

Hazelnut-Crusted Salmon:
Ingredients: Hazelnuts, salmon fillet, lemon, herbs.
Nutritional Intake (per serving): Calories: 260, Omega-3 Fatty Acids, Protein: 20g.

Healthy Fats

Avocado and Salmon Sushi Bowl:
Ingredients: Avocado, salmon, brown rice, seaweed, soy sauce.
Nutritional Intake (per serving): Calories: 300, Healthy Fats, Omega-3 Fatty Acids, Protein: 25g.

Mediterranean Hummus Wrap:
Ingredients: Whole grain wrap, hummus, olive tapenade, tomatoes, cucumbers.
Nutritional Intake (per serving): Calories: 250, Healthy Fats, Fiber: 8g, Protein: 10g.

Olive Oil and Herb Roasted Vegetables:
Ingredients: Mixed vegetables, olive oil, herbs.
Nutritional Intake (per serving): Calories: 180, Healthy Fats, Fiber: 7g.

Walnut and Spinach Salad with Balsamic Vinaigrette:

Ingredients: Walnuts, spinach, cherry tomatoes, feta cheese, balsamic vinaigrette.

Nutritional Intake (per serving): Calories: 220, Healthy Fats, Fiber: 5g.

Coconut Milk and Chickpea Curry:

Ingredients: Chickpeas, coconut milk, tomatoes, curry spices.

Nutritional Intake (per serving): Calories: 280, Healthy Fats, Fiber: 10g, Protein: 12g.

Pesto Zoodles with Pine Nuts:

Ingredients: Zucchini noodles, basil pesto, pine nuts, cherry tomatoes.

Nutritional Intake (per serving): Calories: 230, Healthy Fats, Fiber: 6g.

Almond-Crusted Baked Tilapia:

Ingredients: Almond meal, tilapia fillet, lemon, herbs.

Nutritional Intake (per serving): Calories: 250, Healthy Fats, Protein: 25g.

Cashew and Mango Quinoa Salad:

Ingredients: Quinoa, cashews, mango, red onion, cilantro, lime dressing.

Nutritional Intake (per serving): Calories: 280, Healthy Fats, Fiber: 8g, Protein: 10g.

Flaxseed and Berry Smoothie:
Ingredients: Flaxseeds, mixed berries, Greek yogurt, almond milk.
Nutritional Intake (per serving): Calories: 200, Healthy Fats, Fiber: 7g, Protein: 15g.

Hazelnut and Dark Chocolate Energy Bites:
Ingredients: Hazelnuts, dark chocolate, dates, cocoa powder.
Nutritional Intake (per serving): Calories: 180, Healthy Fats, Fiber: 4g, Protein: 5g.

Eggs

Vegetable Omelette:
Ingredients: Eggs, bell peppers, tomatoes, spinach, feta cheese.
Nutritional Intake (per serving): Calories: 200, Protein: 15g, Healthy Fats.

Avocado and Egg Toast:
Ingredients: Whole grain toast, avocado, poached egg, cherry tomatoes.
Nutritional Intake (per serving): Calories: 250, Protein: 12g, Healthy Fats.

Mushroom and Spinach Egg Muffins:
Ingredients: Eggs, mushrooms, spinach, low-fat cheese.
Nutritional Intake (per serving): Calories: 180, Protein: 15g, Healthy Fats.

Smoked Salmon and Asparagus Frittata:
Ingredients: Eggs, smoked salmon, asparagus, dill.
Nutritional Intake (per serving): Calories: 220, Protein: 20g, Omega-3 Fatty Acids.

Greek Yogurt Deviled Eggs:
Ingredients: Hard-boiled eggs, Greek yogurt, mustard, chives.
Nutritional Intake (per serving): Calories: 160, Protein: 12g, Healthy Fats.

Sweet Potato and Kale Hash with Eggs:
Ingredients: Sweet potatoes, kale, eggs, olive oil.
Nutritional Intake (per serving): Calories: 230, Protein: 15g, Fiber: 6g.

Egg and Vegetable Stir-Fry:
Ingredients: Eggs, mixed vegetables, soy sauce, ginger.
Nutritional Intake (per serving): Calories: 190, Protein: 14g, Healthy Fats.

Caprese Egg Salad:
Ingredients: Hard-boiled eggs, cherry tomatoes, fresh mozzarella, basil, balsamic glaze.
Nutritional Intake (per serving): Calories: 220, Protein: 15g, Healthy Fats.

Spinach and Feta Egg Muffins:
Ingredients: Eggs, spinach, feta cheese, cherry tomatoes.
Nutritional Intake (per serving): Calories: 180, Protein: 14g, Healthy Fats.

Egg and Quinoa Breakfast Bowl:
Ingredients: Eggs, cooked quinoa, avocado, salsa.
Nutritional Intake (per serving): Calories: 250, Protein: 18g, Healthy Fats.

Fish

Grilled Salmon with Lemon and Dill:
Ingredients: Salmon fillet, lemon, dill, olive oil.
Nutritional Intake (per serving): Calories: 250, Omega-3 Fatty Acids, Protein: 25g.

Baked Cod with Tomato and Olive Salsa:
Ingredients: Cod fillet, cherry tomatoes, olives, garlic, olive oil.
Nutritional Intake (per serving): Calories: 220, Omega-3 Fatty Acids, Protein: 20g.

Tuna and Avocado Salad:
Ingredients: Canned tuna, avocado, cherry tomatoes, mixed greens.
Nutritional Intake (per serving): Calories: 230, Omega-3 Fatty Acids, Protein: 15g.

Miso Glazed Halibut:
Ingredients: Halibut fillet, miso paste, soy sauce, ginger.
Nutritional Intake (per serving): Calories: 200, Omega-3 Fatty Acids, Protein: 22g.

Lemon Garlic Shrimp Stir-Fry:
Ingredients: Shrimp, broccoli, bell peppers, garlic, lemon.
Nutritional Intake (per serving): Calories: 180, Omega-3 Fatty Acids, Protein: 20g.

Grilled Mahi-Mahi Tacos:
Ingredients: Mahi-mahi fillets, whole grain tortillas, cabbage slaw, lime crema.
Nutritional Intake (per serving): Calories: 280, Omega-3 Fatty Acids, Protein: 25g.

Baked Rainbow Trout with Herbs:
Ingredients: Rainbow trout, herbs (parsley, thyme), lemon, olive oil.
Nutritional Intake (per serving): Calories: 210, Omega-3 Fatty Acids, Protein: 22g.

Salmon and Quinoa Stuffed Bell Peppers:
Ingredients: Salmon, quinoa, bell peppers, tomatoes, herbs.
Nutritional Intake (per serving): Calories: 260, Omega-3 Fatty Acids, Protein: 25g.

Cilantro-Lime Grilled Swordfish:
Ingredients: Swordfish steaks, cilantro, lime, garlic, olive oil.
Nutritional Intake (per serving): Calories: 240, Omega-3 Fatty Acids, Protein: 28g.

Baked Sardines with Mediterranean Salsa:
Ingredients: Sardines, cherry tomatoes, olives, capers, parsley.
Nutritional Intake (per serving): Calories: 190, Omega-3 Fatty Acids, Protein: 20g.

Limited sodium

Herb-Roasted Chicken Breast:
Ingredients: Chicken breast, garlic, rosemary, thyme, olive oil.
Nutritional Intake (per serving): Calories: 200, Sodium: 80mg, Protein: 25g.

Quinoa and Vegetable Stir-Fry:
Ingredients: Quinoa, broccoli, bell peppers, soy sauce (low-sodium), ginger.
Nutritional Intake (per serving): Calories: 220, Sodium: 100mg, Protein: 10g.

Salmon and Asparagus Foil Packets:
Ingredients: Salmon fillet, asparagus, lemon, dill, olive oil.
Nutritional Intake (per serving): Calories: 250, Sodium: 90mg, Omega-3 Fatty Acids, Protein: 25g.

Mango and Black Bean Salad:
Ingredients: Black beans, mango, red onion, cilantro, lime juice.
Nutritional Intake (per serving): Calories: 180, Sodium: 80mg, Fiber: 8g.

Turkey and Veggie Lettuce Wraps:
Ingredients: Ground turkey, lettuce leaves, bell peppers, garlic, low-sodium soy sauce.
Nutritional Intake (per serving): Calories: 220, Sodium: 120mg, Protein: 20g.

Baked Cod with Lemon and Herbs:
Ingredients: Cod fillet, lemon, parsley, olive oil.
Nutritional Intake (per serving): Calories: 190, Sodium: 100mg, Protein: 22g.

Egg White Omelette with Spinach and Tomatoes:
Ingredients: Egg whites, spinach, tomatoes, herbs.
Nutritional Intake (per serving): Calories: 150, Sodium: 80mg, Protein: 15g.

Cauliflower Rice and Vegetable Bowl:
Ingredients: Cauliflower rice, mixed vegetables, garlic, low-sodium vegetable broth.
Nutritional Intake (per serving): Calories: 170, Sodium: 90mg, Fiber: 6g.

Lentil and Vegetable Soup:
Ingredients: Lentils, carrots, celery, tomatoes, low-sodium vegetable broth.
Nutritional Intake (per serving): Calories: 160, Sodium: 80mg, Fiber: 10g.

Greek Yogurt and Berry Parfait:
Ingredients: Greek yogurt, mixed berries, almonds, honey.
Nutritional Intake (per serving): Calories: 180, Sodium: 50mg, Protein: 15g.

Limited Added sugar

Berry and Greek Yogurt Smoothie:
Ingredients: Mixed berries, Greek yogurt, almond milk, chia seeds.
Nutritional Intake (per serving): Calories: 180, Added Sugar: 0g, Protein: 15g.

Baked Apples with Cinnamon and Walnuts:
Ingredients: Apples, cinnamon, walnuts, a drizzle of honey (optional).
Nutritional Intake (per serving): Calories: 150, Added Sugar: 2g, Fiber: 5g.

Chia Seed Pudding with Fresh Fruit:
Ingredients: Chia seeds, almond milk, vanilla extract, fresh fruit.
Nutritional Intake (per serving): Calories: 200, Added Sugar: 0g, Fiber: 8g.

Sweet Potato and Black Bean Quinoa Bowl:
Ingredients: Quinoa, sweet potatoes, black beans, avocado, lime.
Nutritional Intake (per serving): Calories: 250, Added Sugar: 0g, Fiber: 10g.

Grilled Pineapple with Mint:
Ingredients: Pineapple slices, fresh mint, a sprinkle of cinnamon.
Nutritional Intake (per serving): Calories: 120, Added Sugar: 0g.

Cucumber and Watermelon Salad:
Ingredients: Cucumbers, watermelon, feta cheese, mint, balsamic glaze.
Nutritional Intake (per serving): Calories: 100, Added Sugar: 0g, Protein: 4g.

Oatmeal with Berries and Nuts:
Ingredients: Rolled oats, mixed berries, almonds, a drizzle of maple syrup (optional).
Nutritional Intake (per serving): Calories: 220, Added Sugar: 3g, Fiber: 6g.

Roasted Brussels Sprouts with Balsamic Glaze:

Ingredients: Brussels sprouts, balsamic vinegar, olive oil.

Nutritional Intake (per serving): Calories: 120, Added Sugar: 0g, Fiber: 6g.

Hummus and Veggie Snack Platter:

Ingredients: Hummus, cucumber, carrots, cherry tomatoes.

Nutritional Intake (per serving): Calories: 180, Added Sugar: 0g, Protein: 6g.

Almond Butter and Banana Sandwich:

Ingredients: Whole grain bread, almond butter, banana slices.

Nutritional Intake (per serving): Calories: 250, Added Sugar: 0g, Protein: 8g.

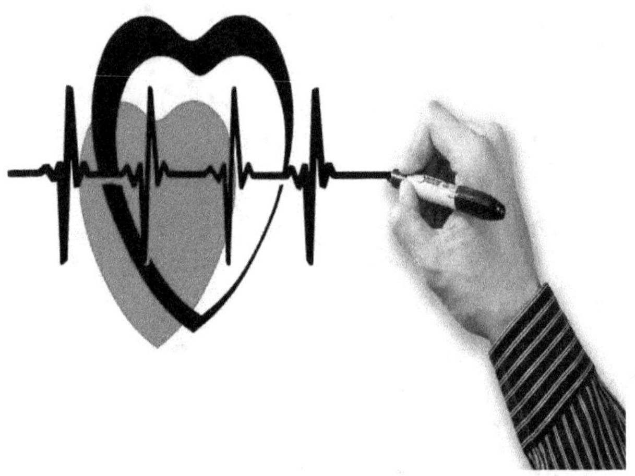

Breakfast Recipes

Greek Yogurt Parfait:
Ingredients: Greek yogurt, mixed berries, almonds, honey.
Nutritional Intake (per serving): Calories: 200, Protein: 15g, Fiber: 5g.

Oatmeal with Chia Seeds and Fresh Fruit:
Ingredients: Rolled oats, chia seeds, almond milk, sliced bananas, strawberries.
Nutritional Intake (per serving): Calories: 250, Protein: 7g, Fiber: 10g.

Whole Grain Avocado Toast:
Ingredients: Whole grain bread, avocado, cherry tomatoes, a sprinkle of feta cheese.
Nutritional Intake (per serving): Calories: 220, Healthy Fats, Fiber: 8g.

Spinach and Feta Egg White Omelette:
Ingredients: Egg whites, spinach, feta cheese, tomatoes.
Nutritional Intake (per serving): Calories: 180, Protein: 20g, Healthy Fats.

Smoothie Bowl with Nut Butter and Granola:
Ingredients: Mixed berries, banana, almond milk, nut butter, granola.
Nutritional Intake (per serving): Calories: 280, Protein: 10g, Healthy Fats.

Chia Seed Pudding with Almond Butter:
Ingredients: Chia seeds, almond milk, almond butter, sliced almonds.
Nutritional Intake (per serving): Calories: 220, Protein: 8g, Healthy Fats.

Whole Wheat Pancakes with Berries:
Ingredients: Whole wheat flour, almond milk, berries, maple syrup.
Nutritional Intake (per serving): Calories: 200, Protein: 6g, Fiber: 5g.

Salmon and Avocado Breakfast Wrap:
Ingredients: Smoked salmon, whole grain wrap, avocado, cream cheese.
Nutritional Intake (per serving): Calories: 250, Omega-3 Fatty Acids, Protein: 20g.

Quinoa Breakfast Bowl with Nuts and Fruit:
Ingredients: Cooked quinoa, mixed nuts, diced apples, cinnamon.
Nutritional Intake (per serving): Calories: 230, Protein: 8g, Fiber: 6g.

Baked Sweet Potato with Cottage Cheese and Berries:

Ingredients: Baked sweet potato, cottage cheese, mixed berries.

Nutritional Intake (per serving): Calories: 180, Protein: 15g, Fiber: 4g.

Lunch Recipes

Grilled Chicken Salad with Balsamic Vinaigrette:

Ingredients: Grilled chicken breast, mixed greens, cherry tomatoes, cucumber, balsamic vinaigrette.

Nutritional Intake (per serving): Calories: 300, Protein: 25g, Fiber: 5g.

Quinoa and Vegetable Buddha Bowl:

Ingredients: Quinoa, roasted vegetables (bell peppers, broccoli, carrots), hummus, avocado.

Nutritional Intake (per serving): Calories: 350, Protein: 12g, Fiber: 10g.

Salmon and Avocado Wrap:

Ingredients: Grilled salmon, whole grain wrap, avocado, lettuce, Greek yogurt sauce.

Nutritional Intake (per serving): Calories: 320, Omega-3 Fatty Acids, Protein: 22g.

Mediterranean Chickpea Salad:
Ingredients: Chickpeas, cherry tomatoes, cucumber, feta cheese, olives, olive oil.
Nutritional Intake (per serving): Calories: 280, Protein: 10g, Fiber: 8g.

Vegetarian Quinoa Stuffed Bell Peppers:
Ingredients: Quinoa, black beans, corn, bell peppers, salsa.
Nutritional Intake (per serving): Calories: 240, Protein: 8g, Fiber: 10g.

Tuna and White Bean Salad:
Ingredients: Canned tuna, white beans, cherry tomatoes, red onion, lemon vinaigrette.
Nutritional Intake (per serving): Calories: 260, Protein: 20g, Fiber: 7g.

Whole Wheat Veggie Wrap with Hummus:
Ingredients: Whole wheat wrap, hummus, assorted vegetables, feta cheese.
Nutritional Intake (per serving): Calories: 280, Protein: 12g, Fiber: 8g.

Lemon Garlic Shrimp and Quinoa Bowl:
Ingredients: Shrimp, quinoa, broccoli, lemon, garlic.
Nutritional Intake (per serving): Calories: 310, Protein: 25g, Fiber: 7g.

Turkey and Spinach Stuffed Portobello Mushrooms:
Ingredients: Ground turkey, spinach, Portobello mushrooms, feta cheese.
Nutritional Intake (per serving): Calories: 230, Protein: 18g, Fiber: 5g.

Vegan Lentil Soup:
Ingredients: Lentils, carrots, celery, tomatoes, vegetable broth, spices.
Nutritional Intake (per serving): Calories: 220, Protein: 15g, Fiber: 10g.

Dinner Recipes

Grilled Salmon with Lemon-Dill Sauce:
Ingredients: Grilled salmon fillet, lemon-dill sauce, steamed asparagus, quinoa.
Nutritional Intake (per serving): Calories: 350, Omega-3 Fatty Acids, Protein: 30g.

Vegetarian Chickpea and Spinach Curry:
Ingredients: Chickpeas, spinach, tomatoes, coconut milk, brown rice.
Nutritional Intake (per serving): Calories: 320, Protein: 15g, Fiber: 10g.

Baked Chicken Breast with Roasted Vegetables:

Ingredients: Baked chicken breast, mixed roasted vegetables (sweet potatoes, Brussels sprouts, carrots), olive oil.

Nutritional Intake (per serving): Calories: 300, Protein: 25g, Fiber: 8g.

Mushroom and Lentil Stuffed Bell Peppers:

Ingredients: Lentils, mushrooms, bell peppers, tomatoes, quinoa.

Nutritional Intake (per serving): Calories: 280, Protein: 18g, Fiber: 9g.

Whole Wheat Pasta with Tomato and Basil Sauce:

Ingredients: Whole wheat pasta, fresh tomato-basil sauce, grilled chicken, broccoli.

Nutritional Intake (per serving): Calories: 320, Protein: 20g, Fiber: 10g.

Tofu Stir-Fry with Brown Rice:

Ingredients: Tofu, mixed vegetables, soy sauce, ginger, brown rice.

Nutritional Intake (per serving): Calories: 300, Protein: 15g, Fiber: 8g.

Lemon Herb Baked Cod:
Ingredients: Baked cod fillet, lemon, herbs, quinoa, steamed green beans.
Nutritional Intake (per serving): Calories: 280, Protein: 25g, Fiber: 7g.

Veggie and Quinoa Stuffed Acorn Squash:
Ingredients: Quinoa, acorn squash, mixed vegetables, feta cheese.
Nutritional Intake (per serving): Calories: 250, Protein: 10g, Fiber: 8g.

Shrimp and Vegetable Skewers:
Ingredients: Grilled shrimp, bell peppers, onions, cherry tomatoes, whole grain couscous.
Nutritional Intake (per serving): Calories: 290, Protein: 20g, Fiber: 6g.

Black Bean and Sweet Potato Chili:
Ingredients: Black beans, sweet potatoes, tomatoes, chili spices, avocado.
Nutritional Intake (per serving): Calories: 280, Protein: 12g, Fiber: 10g.

Mixed Berry Parfait:
Ingredients: Mixed berries, Greek yogurt, granola.
Nutritional Intake (per serving): Calories: 150, Protein: 8g, Fiber: 5g.

Dark Chocolate-Dipped Strawberries:
Ingredients: Fresh strawberries, dark chocolate (70% cocoa or higher).
Nutritional Intake (per serving): Calories: 100, Antioxidants.

Chia Seed and Mango Pudding:
Ingredients: Chia seeds, almond milk, ripe mango.
Nutritional Intake (per serving): Calories: 180, Fiber: 8g, Omega-3 Fatty Acids.

Baked Apples with Cinnamon and Walnuts:
Ingredients: Apples, cinnamon, walnuts.
Nutritional Intake (per serving): Calories: 120, Fiber: 4g.

Frozen Banana and Peanut Butter Bites:
Ingredients: Sliced bananas, natural peanut butter.
Nutritional Intake (per serving): Calories: 150, Protein: 4g, Healthy Fats.

Yogurt and Berry Popsicles:
Ingredients: Greek yogurt, mixed berries, honey.
Nutritional Intake (per serving): Calories: 120,
Protein: 5g.

Oatmeal and Date Energy Balls:
Ingredients: Rolled oats, dates, almond butter.
Nutritional Intake (per serving): Calories: 160,
Fiber: 4g.

Coconut and Berry Chia Seed Popsicles:
Ingredients: Coconut milk, mixed berries, chia
seeds.
Nutritional Intake (per serving): Calories: 130,
Fiber: 5g, Healthy Fats.

Avocado Chocolate Mousse:
Ingredients: Avocado, cocoa powder, honey.
Nutritional Intake (per serving): Calories: 180,
Healthy Fats, Fiber: 6g.

Peach and Almond Crisp:
Ingredients: Fresh peaches, almond flour, oats,
cinnamon.
Nutritional Intake (per serving): Calories: 200,
Fiber: 5g, Healthy Fats.

Almond Butter and Banana Slices:
Ingredients: Banana slices, almond butter.
Nutritional Intake (per serving): Calories: 150,
Protein: 4g, Healthy Fats.

Greek Yogurt with Berries and Nuts:
Ingredients: Greek yogurt, mixed berries,
almonds.
Nutritional Intake (per serving): Calories: 180,
Protein: 15g, Healthy Fats.

Hummus and Veggie Sticks:
Ingredients: Hummus, carrot and cucumber
sticks.
Nutritional Intake (per serving): Calories: 120,
Protein: 5g, Fiber: 6g.

Trail Mix with Dried Fruits and Nuts:
Ingredients: Almonds, walnuts, dried
cranberries, dark chocolate chips.
Nutritional Intake (per serving): Calories: 200,
Protein: 6g, Healthy Fats.

Cottage Cheese and Pineapple Cubes:
Ingredients: Cottage cheese, fresh pineapple
cubes.
Nutritional Intake (per serving): Calories: 160,
Protein: 15g, Vitamin C.

Whole Grain Crackers with Avocado:
Ingredients: Whole grain crackers, sliced avocado, cherry tomatoes.
Nutritional Intake (per serving): Calories: 180, Healthy Fats, Fiber: 5g.

Roasted Chickpeas:
Ingredients: Chickpeas, olive oil, spices.
Nutritional Intake (per serving): Calories: 150, Protein: 6g, Fiber: 5g.

Apple Slices with Nut Butter:
Ingredients: Apple slices, almond butter or peanut butter.
Nutritional Intake (per serving): Calories: 160, Protein: 3g, Healthy Fats.

Yogurt and Berry Parfait:
Ingredients: Low-fat yogurt, mixed berries, granola.
Nutritional Intake (per serving): Calories: 200, Protein: 10g, Fiber: 4g.

Vegetable and Guacamole Dip:
Ingredients: Sliced bell peppers, cherry tomatoes, guacamole.
Nutritional Intake (per serving): Calories: 140, Healthy Fats, Vitamin C.

Smoothies Recipes

Berry Blast Smoothie:
Ingredients: Mixed berries (strawberries, blueberries, raspberries), Greek yogurt, almond milk, chia seeds.
Nutritional Intake (per serving): Calories: 200, Protein: 10g, Fiber: 8g.

Green Power Smoothie:
Ingredients: Spinach, kale, banana, pineapple, almond milk.
Nutritional Intake (per serving): Calories: 180, Vitamin C, Fiber: 7g.

Tropical Paradise Smoothie:
Ingredients: Mango, pineapple, coconut water, Greek yogurt.
Nutritional Intake (per serving): Calories: 220, Vitamin C, Protein: 12g.

Avocado and Banana Smoothie:
Ingredients: Avocado, banana, spinach, almond milk, honey.
Nutritional Intake (per serving): Calories: 250, Healthy Fats, Fiber: 9g.

Chocolate-Berry Protein Smoothie:
Ingredients: Mixed berries, chocolate protein powder, almond milk, chia seeds.
Nutritional Intake (per serving): Calories: 230, Protein: 20g, Fiber: 6g.

Peach and Oatmeal Smoothie:
Ingredients: Peaches, rolled oats, low-fat yogurt, almond milk.
Nutritional Intake (per serving): Calories: 220, Fiber: 8g, Protein: 9g.

Cherry Almond Spinach Smoothie:
Ingredients: Cherries, almonds, spinach, Greek yogurt, coconut water.
Nutritional Intake (per serving): Calories: 240, Protein: 14g, Healthy Fats.

Pineapple Mint Cucumber Smoothie:
Ingredients: Pineapple, cucumber, mint leaves, lime, coconut water.
Nutritional Intake (per serving): Calories: 160, Vitamin C, Fiber: 5g.

Blueberry and Kale Protein Smoothie:
Ingredients: Blueberries, kale, protein powder, almond milk.
Nutritional Intake (per serving): Calories: 210, Protein: 18g, Fiber: 7g.

Mango Ginger Turmeric Smoothie:
Ingredients: Mango, ginger, turmeric, plain yogurt, orange juice.
Nutritional Intake (per serving): Calories: 190, Vitamin C, Anti-Inflammatory.

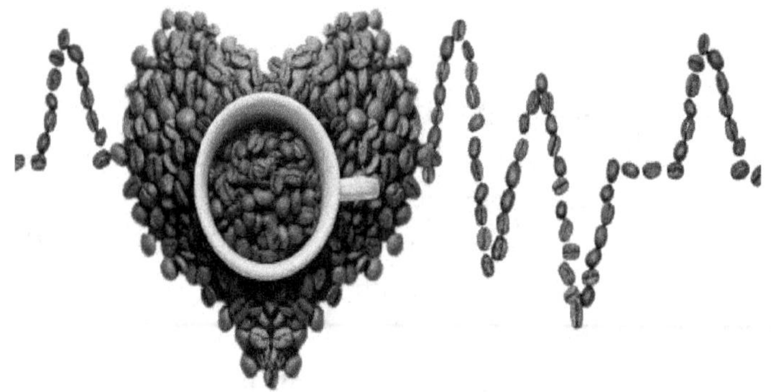

SHOPPING LIST

1. Fruits:
- Apples
- Bananas
- Berries (strawberries, blueberries, raspberries)
- Oranges
- Grapes
- Pineapple
- Mangoes
- Kiwi
- Pomegranates
- Watermelon

2. Vegetables:
- Spinach
- Kale
- Broccoli
- Brussels sprouts
- Bell peppers
- Carrots
- Tomatoes
- Avocado
- Sweet potatoes
- Zucchini

3. Whole Grains:

- Quinoa
- Brown rice
- Oats
- Barley
- Whole wheat bread
- Whole grain pasta
- Bulgur
- Farro
- Buckwheat
- Millet

4. Lean Proteins:

- Chicken breast
- Turkey breast
- Salmon
- Tuna
- Cod
- Lentils
- Chickpeas
- Black beans
- Tofu
- Greek yogurt

5. Nuts and Seeds:

- Almonds
- Walnuts
- Chia seeds
- Flaxseeds

- Sunflower seeds
- Pumpkin seeds
- Pistachios
- Cashews
- Pecans
- Hemp seeds

6. Dairy and Dairy Alternatives:
- Low-fat or fat-free milk
- Greek yogurt
- Cottage cheese
- Almond milk
- Soy milk
- Coconut milk (unsweetened)
- Feta cheese
- Parmesan cheese (in moderation)

7. Healthy Fats:
- Olive oil
- Avocado oil
- Flaxseed oil
- Canola oil
- Avocado
- Olives
- Fatty fish (salmon, mackerel, trout)
- Chia seeds
- Walnuts

8. Herbs and Spices:

- Garlic
- Turmeric
- Cinnamon
- Ginger
- Oregano
- Basil
- Rosemary
- Thyme
- Cumin
- Paprika

9. Beverages:

- Green tea
- Herbal tea
- Water (plain or infused with fruits)
- Coffee (in moderation)

10. Whole Foods Snacks:

- Air-popped popcorn
- Rice cakes
- Hummus with carrot or cucumber sticks
- Greek yogurt with berries
- Dark chocolate (in moderation)

CONCLUSION

In the intricate weaving of promoting heart health, the Heart Healthy Foods Chart emerges as a beacon of guidance and empowerment. As we conclude this insightful journey through nutrient-rich choices and mindful dietary selections, it becomes evident that the path to a healthy heart is paved with conscious and informed decisions.

The Heart Healthy Foods Chart encapsulates the wisdom of incorporating a diverse array of fruits, vegetables, whole grains, lean proteins, and heart-friendly fats into our daily meals. By offering a visual representation of wholesome choices, it serves as a practical tool to simplify the complexities of nutrition, enabling individuals to make choices aligned with their cardiovascular well-being.

This chart is more than a mere compilation of food items; it is a testament to the profound connection between what we eat and the resilience of our hearts. It encourages a holistic approach to nourishment, emphasizing the importance of balance, moderation, and a keen understanding of the impact of dietary choices on our cardiovascular system.

As we embrace the principles outlined in the Heart Healthy Foods Chart, we embark on a journey towards sustained heart wellness. By incorporating these principles into our daily lives, we not only fortify our cardiovascular health but also lay the foundation for a vibrant and fulfilling existence. Let this chart be a constant reminder that every meal is an opportunity to nourish our hearts and cultivate a resilient, thriving life. Armed with the knowledge within this chart, we stride confidently towards a heart-healthy future—one plate at a time.

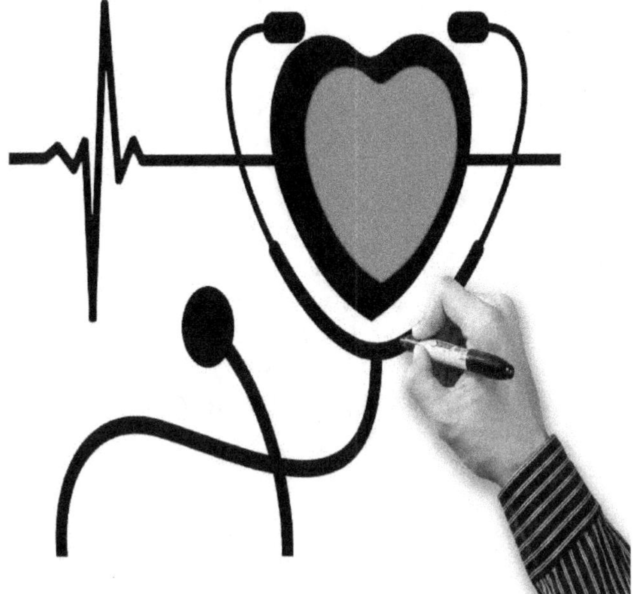